Asthma

I0146101

Asthma Cure
How To Treat Asthma
How To Prevent Asthma
All Natural Remedies For Asthma
Medical Breakthroughs For Asthma
And Proper Diet And Exercise For Asthma

By Ace McCloud
Copyright © 2014

Disclaimer

The information provided in this book is designed to provide helpful information on the subjects discussed. This book is not meant to be used, nor should it be used, to diagnose or treat any medical condition. For diagnosis or treatment of any medical problem, consult your own physician. The publisher and author are not responsible for any specific health or allergy needs that may require medical supervision and are not liable for any damages or negative consequences from any treatment, action, application or preparation, to any person reading or following the information in this book. Any references included are provided for informational purposes only. Readers should be aware that any websites or links listed in this book may change.

Table of Contents

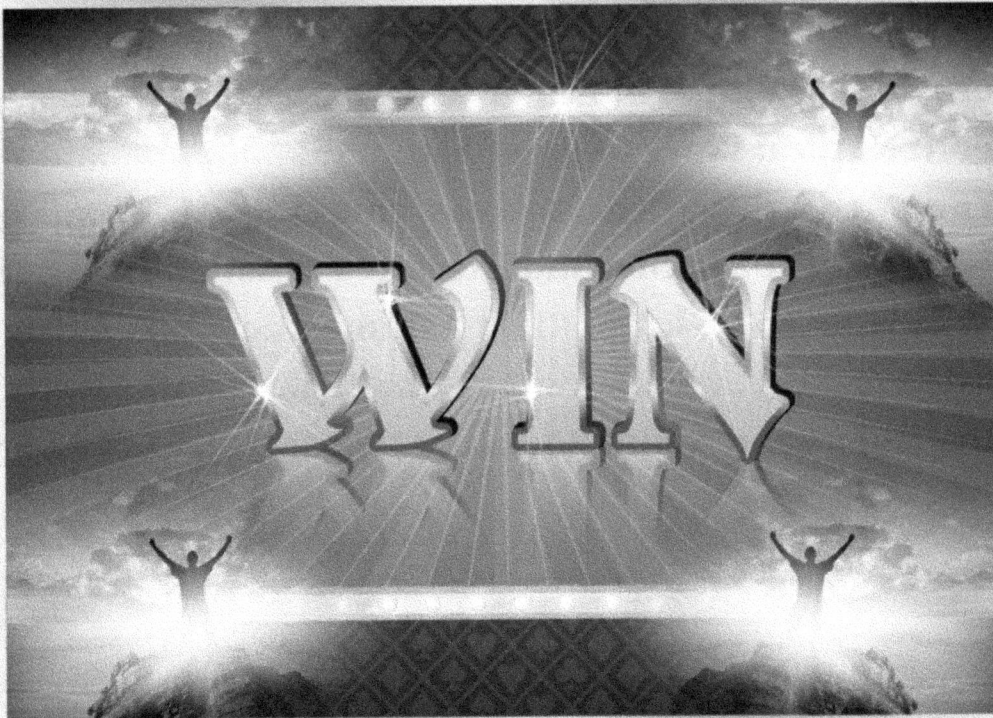

DEDICATED TO THOSE WHO ARE PLAYING THE GAME OF LIFE TO

WIN

KEEP ON PUSHING AND NEVER GIVE UP!

Ace McCloud

Be sure to check out my website for all my Books and Audio books.

www.AcesEbooks.com

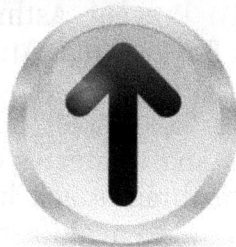

Introduction

I want to thank you and congratulate you for buying the book, "Asthma Cure: How To Treat Asthma, How To Prevent Asthma, All Natural Remedies For Asthma, Medical Breakthroughs For Asthma, And Proper Diet And Exercise For Asthma".

This book contains proven steps and strategies on how to control your asthma symptoms over time and if an asthma attack happens. In this book you will discover what triggers asthma, how to avoid asthma attacks, and how to make simple changes in your environment to eliminate as many triggers as possible. It also aims to help you become more familiar with the best natural and medical options for treating asthma, both over-the-counter and by prescription. You will also discover how to enhance your diet with asthma-friendly foods and how to get in plenty of exercise without triggering an asthma attack, including how to learn special breathing exercises. Finally, this book aims to help you learn what you need to know when picking an asthma specialist. Stop suffering today and enjoy your life, no matter how severe your asthma is. It's time to breathe easier!

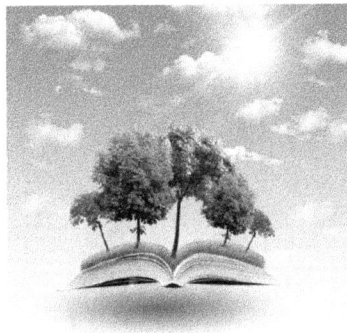

Chapter 1: What is Asthma?

At least 25 million people around the world suffer from asthma—it effects both children and adults. Asthma is a chronic disease and is not curable. It is a lung disease that causes your lungs to become inflamed. When your lungs become inflamed, your airways become narrow and it causes you to have trouble breathing. Your airways are what carry oxygen to your lungs to help you breathe. People who suffer from asthma incur a swelling in their airways. Their airways become very sensitive to certain substances when inhaled and can tighten up, making it harder for oxygen to pass in and out of their lungs.

Although many people develop asthma during childhood, it is very possible to develop it at some point when you're an adult. The most common symptoms of asthma include a tightness in the chest, a shortness of breath, late night/early morning coughing, wheezing, increased mucus, and uncomfortable breathing. Symptoms of asthma vary in their intensity and frequency and its effects can fluctuate in a single person over time. While some people suffer from mild asthma, some people suffer from severe asthma, and some people only have asthma attacks after exercising. No two cases of asthma are the same. Many doctors believe that the cause of asthma is linked to people's genes and their environmental factors. For example, if asthma is relevant in your family history, you probably have increased chances of developing it as well. Also, environmental factors such as cockroaches, cigarette and wood smoke, exhaust, farm animals, pesticides, and certain pets are known to aggravate symptoms of asthma.

While asthma in some people is mild and will go away on its own with just a little medicine, some people can have very severe cases that need special attention. When a person begins to show symptoms from severe asthma, they are essentially having an asthma attack, also known as a flareup. Asthma attacks can be fatal and require urgent care. Although asthma can be treated with medicine, there is no cure for the disease itself. Even if you have it and feel fine one day, it can flareup at any given time.

Those who suffer from asthma also tend to experience a harder lifestyle. Since asthma generally gets worse at night and in the early morning, it is very hard to sleep peacefully, especially when you're having a flareup. It can cause you to miss work and school and it can cause you to limit the amount of time you spend exercising. Poorly controlling your asthma can also be very costly—if you do not take care of it, you can end up having more doctors office and emergency room visits and you will have to pay for extra medications that your insurance may not cover. The good news is that as long as you keep your asthma under control, you can still enjoy a cost-effective, healthy, normal lifestyle.

As you read on, you will learn how to live a normal life, despite your asthma condition. You will read about the different ways to treat asthma by eliminating triggers and using home remedies. You will learn about some of the best natural supplements that can reduce your asthma symptoms as well as some of the best modern medical practices to treat asthma. You will learn about some of the best "asthma-friendly" foods to add to your diet as well as the best types of exercise for your lungs. You will learn about different yoga positions and breathing exercises that can help you with your breathing. All in all, the book aims to be the ultimate guide to helping you live a positive, happy life while easily managing your asthma.

Chapter 2: Controlling Your Asthma

Although doctors are unsure of the main reason why people develop asthma, it is true that you have a higher chance of developing it if it runs in your family. Unfortunately, there is not much you can do to protect yourself from developing it at all. However, if you do develop it, there are some things you can do to help yourself keep it under control.

By knowing what sets your asthma off, you can begin to take preventative measures against it. Those who already suffer from asthma must take steps to avoid asthma triggers, which are things that can aggravate your asthma symptoms. Some common examples of asthma triggers are air smog, allergies, cold air, cold or flu viruses, sinusitis, smoke, and certain fragrances. Asthma triggers generally vary from person to person—for example, what triggers one person's asthma may not trigger your asthma.

One great way to figure out what your asthma triggers are is to keep a journal or a record. Take a special notebook and keep track of when your symptoms are aggravated, what time of day it was, what environmental factors may have contributed to it, and what you were doing when it happened. Over time, you will be able to identify a pattern or patterns of what sets off your asthma. When you've figured this out, you can make changes in your lifestyle and environment to eliminate those triggers. This chapter will go over some of the most common triggers to help you reduce your chances of having an asthma attack.

Keeping Allergies Under Control

If you suffer from allergies in addition to asthma, you may need to see an allergies specialist to determine if your allergies are aggravating your asthma symptoms. A specialist will be able to quickly identify any substances that you are allergic too, which you can then eliminate from your environment or diet to reduce the chances of an asthma attack. 25% of people develop allergies at so during the course of their lives, so it is important to be aware of what you are allergic too, especially when trying to manage your asthma.

Dust Mites and Mold Allergies

Two of the most common home-environment allergies are caused by dust mites and mold. Dust mites can easily induce an asthma attack because they are often found in your bedding, which you probably use every day. Luckily, you can take some simple steps to reduce the amount of dust mites that appear in your home. You can invest in a special dust mite cover for your pillows and mattress. One of the best products for preventing dust mites in your pillows is the Allersoft 100% Cotton Dust Mite Pillow Encasement. This pillow cover is an excellent defense against dust mites, pet dander, and other allergens that can aggravate your asthma symptoms. A great mattress cover is the Luna Premium Mattress Protector. This mattress cover will protect you from dust mites and allergens and is 100% hypoallergenic. It is specially designed for those who suffer from asthma and it comes with a 10 year warranty, should anything go wrong.

Additionally, you should also wash all of your pillow cases, sheets, and blankets in hot water every week and vacuum two times per week. Also invest in curtains that are washable as well. If you do not have hardwood floors, buy carpeting that can be washed and try to stay away from throw rugs. Make sure you keep your environment free of clutter and make sure that you consistently dust all of your surfaces.

Finally, a dehumidifier will help you keep the humidity of your home low. There are many different kinds of dehumidifiers available to buy. For small spaces such as your closet, a washing machine, or your bathroom, one of the greatest and cheapest (but very effective) dehumidifiers is the E-333 Wireless Mini Dehumidifier. This dehumidifier is small, inexpensive, wireless, safe, and has a ten-year lifespan. For larger areas of your home, I highly recommend the Frigidaire 70-pint Dehumidifier. This dehumidifier is larger than the E-333 Wireless Mini Dehumidifier but it eliminates bacteria from the air in your home, protects it from mold and mildew, and can affect a space as large as up to 1400 square feet. Its electronic controls can help you save time and money.

To reduce the chances of mold aggravating your asthma, a dehumidifier can also be of help. Be sure to keep your bathrooms free of carpeting and to clean them regularly, including your shower curtain and floor. You should also regularly clean your basement, garage, crawlspaces, or any other area of your home where mold generally grows. Do not keep indoor plants in your bedrooms and do not store damp clothing unless it is aired out. Never leave wet laundry in your washing machine, either. Mold will quickly grow on anything that is damp and dark. When cleaning mold or looking for mold, be sure to wear a protective dust mask.

Cockroach Allergies

Cockroaches cause another allergy that can worsen your asthma symptoms. Even the cleanest of homes can attract cockroaches and other insects that may affect your asthma. However, there are some steps that you can take to ensure that your home stays clean and free from cockroaches. One of the easiest ways to do this is to lay down cockroach traps. One of the traps that have worked best for me is the Trapper Insect Trap. This product comes with 90 traps and is great for catching cockroaches as well as other pests. They are glue traps, which are non-toxic and great for determining whether you have a large infestation that needs professional attention. Cockroach sprays are also great but should only be used when nobody is home. Also be sure to fix any water leaks and to keep your kitchen clean. Since cockroaches are attracted to food, be sure to keep all food tightly packed and stored away.

Pet Allergies

Finally, many people are allergic to their pets, due to the dander that is found in their fur. If you are already allergic to pet dander, it may be wise not to get a pet that you are allergic too. However, it is possible to develop pet dander allergies after you have gotten a pet. If possible, restrict your pet to a certain area of your home, preferably an area with limited carpeting, or have it live outside. Do not let it stay in your bedroom and keep it washed regularly. If you do not have a pet but your friends or family members do, avoid staying at their homes for a long time to help ease your allergies. One really great product for eliminating pet dander in your home is the Pet CleanAir Tabletop Air Purifier. This device is small, inexpensive, and perfect for the area of your home in which your pet stays. It works very well and collects almost all pet dander that gets into the air. It is perfect for those who have asthma that is worsened by pet dander.

Keep the Rest of Your Body Healthy

A common cold or the flu is a surefire way to aggravate your asthma symptoms. Try to avoid contact with anyone who is sick and wash your hands after touching money or anything else that another person has handled. Also try to maintain a healthy and balanced diet and stick to a committed exercise regime to keep your immune system in tact. While I will get into the proper diet and exercise in the next few chapters, I highly recommend checking out some of my other books to help supplement your general health. If your asthma constantly stresses you out, that stress could start to take a negative toll on your body and health. As you can see, although asthma is not curable, it is definitely treatable, so there is no reason to let it stress you out. To make your life a little happier and lighter, you can check out my book Laughter and Humor Therapy. To learn how to keep your body as healthy and energetic as possible, I also recommend checking out Ultimate Energy.

Taking Additional Steps to Prevent Asthma Attacks

No matter if you are out in public or at home, there are several other steps that you can take to avoid aggravating your asthma symptoms. For example, cigarette smoke is a primary trigger of asthma, so if possible, do not allow others to smoke in your home and ask your friends not to smoke around you, and obviously, don't smoke yourself. Back in the day, you used to have to avoid public places that allowed smoking, such as restaurants, but steps have been taken to ban smoking in many public places. If you are a smoker yourself, it is crucial to try and stop, otherwise you will make your asthma worse. If you need extra help kicking the habit, be sure to reference to my book Quit Smoking Now Quickly and Easily.

At home, try to avoid cleaning with chemicals and use natural substances such as lemon juice and baking soda. Many harsh chemical cleaners contain allergens that can trigger your asthma symptoms. Also, use vent filters on all of the vents in your home. This can help prevent airborne particles that may aggravate your asthma from entering your home. A really good vent filter is the AllerTech Vent

Guard. If possible, see if you can replace all of the flooring in your home with hardwood floors. This option is expensive, so if you are unable to have all hardwood floors in your home, keep your carpeting clean with a good vacuum.

Have an Action Plan

Finally, you should always have a plan on what to do in the event that you do have an asthma attack. Unfortunately, sometimes you cannot prevent a trigger from aggravating your asthma symptoms and if you are unaware of any allergies that you may have, you may not be able to take the necessary steps to prevent them. An action plan should have a set of written instructions that includes what kind of medicines you take, what your triggers are, and what you should do if your symptoms are getting worse. By having an action plan, you will be comfortable and familiar on what to do when you feel an asthma attack coming on. It is almost similar to having a fire drill. It can reduce your chances of having to go to the hospital and it will save you money. Your plan should be updated at least once a year and you should review it with your doctor.

Chapter 3: Natural Ways to Treat Asthma

Though asthma is a respiratory disease and should ultimately be treated with medicine in the case of an emergency, there are several home remedies that you can practice to help treat your asthma when your symptoms are not severe. Understanding how to identify and eliminate triggers from your environment is one way to naturally treat asthma. However, there are some other methods that you can use to treat your asthma without the use of modern medicine. This chapter will cover some natural supplements that you can take to help lessen the severity of your asthma symptoms.

Magnesium

You can help your body keep your airways open with magnesium. Magnesium has plenty of anti-inflammatory properties, making it a great option for controlling asthma. You can get magnesium by eating foods that contain it or you can take it in the form of a supplement. I highly recommend the Nature Made High Potency Magnesium Softgels. You can take one of these capsules per day with water to keep your body healthy and to help reduce your asthma symptoms.

Peppermint Extract

Peppermint extract can be very effective in relieving asthma symptoms because it can serve as a homemade vaporizer. Bring a pot of fresh water to a boil and add ten drops of peppermint extract. Simmer the combination for an hour and the air in the room can help relieve your asthma symptoms if you're feeling them. One of the top peppermint extract products that I recommend is the Bakto Flavors Natural Pepper Extract. This product is the best value because it comes in a three pack for a low price of $13.

Omega-3 Fatty Acids

Substances that contain omega-3 fatty acids, such as fish, may prevent your airways from becoming inflamed. If you don't like fish, you can take fish oil or flaxseed oil supplements to provide your body with omega-3 fatty acids. One of the best fish oil products is Nature Made Fish Oil and one of the best flaxseed oil products is Nature Made Flaxseed Oil. Both products contain the amount of omega-3 fatty acids that your body needs to prevent inflammation. Each product comes in the form of a soft gel tablet, which you can take with a meal.

Vitamins A, C, and E

These vitamins decrease free radical activity in our bodies, which can cause our airways to become inflamed. One way to ensure that you're getting enough of these vitamins is to eat plenty of healthy foods that contain them. You can also take them in the form of a supplement. A great way to provide your body with each of these vitamins at once is to take a multivitamin. One of the best multivitamins that contain each of these and more is the Kirkland Signature Daily Multivitamin. This multivitamin contains 500 tablets for a low price, so they will be able to last you a while before you have to refill. These vitamins also help with staying healthy, energetic, and productive.

Bromelain

Bromelain is an antioxidant that is found in the stems of pineapples. If you take it without any food, it serves as a strong anti-inflammatory enzyme. One way to easily provide your body with Bromelain is to take it through a natural supplement. My favorite Bromelain supplement is NOW Foods Bromelain. This product is made from a vegetarian formula and is very potent. It may help you reduce inflammation in your airways if you suffer from asthma.

Herbal Supplements

There are several herbal supplements that you can also take to help control your asthma. Many Chinese herbs have been proven useful in treating asthma for years. One great product that contains Chinese herbal remedies is the Ridgecrest Herbal Clearlungs Supplement. This product uses a combination of Chinese herbs to promote easy breathing relieve congestion. It comes in a nice orange flavor and best of all, there are several sizes of this product to choose from. You can try it by buying the 60-count and if it works for you, you can buy it with up to 120 capsules.

For relieving traditional asthma symptoms such as chest tightness, shortness of breath, and wheezing, try Ridgecrest Asthma Clear Homeo and Herbal Asthma Relief. This product also utilizes traditional Chinese medicine to treat dry conditions such as wheezing. This product is aimed at providing short-term and long-term relief by opening your lungs.

Another Chinese herb that is great for treating asthma is Reishi Mushroom. This herb has powerful anti-inflammatory properties and helps your lungs become strong. This herb has been used for the last 2,000 years. The mushrooms themselves can be cooked in foods but you can also get this herb in the form of a supplement. One of the best Reishi Mushroom supplements is Nature's Way Reishi Extract. Women who are pregnant should not take this supplement.

There is also a herbal supplement called Black Seed, which can help treat respiratory conditions and lung health. People living in Asia and the Middle East have been using it for thousands of years. It has anti-inflammatory properties, contains high levels of antioxidants, and helps strengthen your immune system, all of which are useful in treating asthma. One of the best black seed products is Amazing Herbs Black Seed.

As always, you should consult with your doctor before taking any herbal medications or before adding a natural supplement to your diet.

Chapter 4: Medical Ways to Treat Asthma

Since asthma is a complex disease, sometimes it is necessary to treat it with modern medication. There are two main purposes the modern medication serves for those who suffer from asthma: to control the disease over time and to help during an attack. Your doctor can help you decide what kinds of modern medications you should take to help your asthma condition. All of the medicine in this chapter that is not indicated as "over-the-counter" will require a doctor's prescription, so you will have to see your doctor to get it. However, this chapter will give you an overview of what you can expect when discussing medical options with your doctor.

Inhalers and Steroids

Inhalers are a form of asthma medicine that helps your airways open when the muscles around them become too tight. They come in the form of a small, portable, easy-to-use device. People often use inhalers to quickly treat chest tightness, a shortness of breath, or wheezing. Inhalers are known as rescue medications so they should not be used every day, only when needed. They are meant to quickly relieve you of any asthma symptoms.

There are two primary types of asthma inhalers: metered dose inhalers and dry power inhalers. A metered dose inhaler has a removable medicine cartridge that you can push on to administer the drug into your lungs. With dry powder inhalers, you must breathe fast and deep to get the drug into your lungs. There are two main types of drugs used in asthma inhalers: anti-inflammatory drugs and bronchodilator drugs. Anti-inflammatory inhalers help reduce swelling and mucus build-up in your airways and can help you in the event of an asthma attack. They are usually best for emergency uses. Many anti-inflammatory inhalers are also steroid inhalers. Bronchodilator inhalers can have short-term or long-term effects and help reduce chest tightness, shortness of breath, and wheezing.

Inhalers and inhaled steroids are safe for kids and adults and generally tend to have little side effects. In some cases, it can cause a yeast infection to develop in your mouth. However, this can easily be managed and preventing by gargling and rinsing your mouth after using an inhaler.

Nebulizers

Nebulizers are similar to inhalers but they utilize a mask or bigger mouthpiece. You can breathe into them normally, making them great options for babies, children or those who are unsure of how to use regular inhalers. Nebulizers provide asthma medication in a mist form instead of liquid form. If you need to take large doses of asthma medication, you can also use a nebulizer. Nebulizers can come in tabletop or portable form, so you can use them almost anywhere. To buy a nebulizer, you will need a prescription from a doctor.

Prednisone

Prednisone is a type of anti-inflammatory steroid asthma medication that is taken orally, enters your bloodstream instead of your lungs, and is for if you have a serious asthma attack. Many doctors prescribe Prednisone to those who have worsening symptoms of asthma. Prednisone can sometimes be an alternative for hospitalization. Your doctor may prescribe you low doses of Prednisone to control your asthma but he or she may also prescribe you multiple high doses for an accelerated effect. Other asthma-related drugs that are similar to Prednisone are Medrol, Deltasone, Prelone, and Decadron. Prednisone and other steroid medications may cause several side effects, including weight gain, bloating, high blood pressure, high blood sugar, growth issues, diabetes, eye cataracts, osteoporosis, and weak muscles.

Theophylline

If you suffer from mild asthma, you can take a medication called Theophylline, which comes in a pill form. This pill works like inhaled steroids because it relaxes your airways and reduces your chances of reacting to a trigger. It can be especially helpful if your asthma gets worse during the night and it is much less of a hassle to take than an inhaled medication. If your doctor decides that Theophylline is right for you, he or she may have you undergo a blood test to make sure that your body is getting enough of the medicine.

Allergy Shots and Medicine

Since allergies are a common trigger for asthma attacks, you may be wondering if an allergy shot can serve as a medical treatment for asthma. This is a relatively new concept known as immunotherapy. One recent study showed that children who received allergy shots had reduced chances of developing asthma and had improved reactions to allergies. You can ask your doctor if an allergy shot can help reduce your asthma symptoms. Your doctor can then refer you to an allergy specialist if needed.

If you would rather take an allergy medication to help relieve your allergy and asthma symptoms, you can try some safe and effective over-the-counter allergy remedies. An over-the-counter decongestant can help dissolve any congestion and help you breathe normally easier, putting less stress on your lungs. A really great decongestant that you can check out is Good Sense Nasal Decongestant. It is comparable to Sudafed, another popular brand of decongestant, is non-drowsy, and works to relieve sinus pressure in addition to congestion. Even if your allergies do not bother you all year, this is a very good product to stock up on for when your allergies do start to bother you.

Another type of over-the-counter allergy medication that you may consider is an expectorant, which helps reduce the amount of mucus that builds up in your airways. A really great expectorant is Kirkland Signature Mucus Relief Chest.

This medicine works to eliminate chest congestion and thins out your mucus, making it easier to cough up. It is comparable to other brands such as Mucinex and Robitussin and works just as great.

Over-the-Counter Asthma Drugs

There are several other over-the-counter drugs that you can buy to treat asthma, although you should not use them to manage your asthma or to keep asthma attacks from happening. The most popular over-the-counter asthma medications is Bronkaid. Over-the-counter asthma medications are meant for quick, emergency asthma solutions and you should consult with your doctor before taking them in case they can cause any side effects. Many people misunderstand the purpose of over-the-counter asthma medication. They are really just designed for emergencies.

Bronchial Thermoplasty

Bronchial Thermoplasty is a relatively simple procedure in which a doctor inserts heated tubes into your airway to help your muscles relax. This procedure is good for adults who suffer from severe asthma. If you are under 18, if you have a pacemaker, or if you are allergic to certain medications, cannot undergo a Bronchial Thermoplasty procedure. 79% of those who underwent this procedure reported having a better quality of life and saw reductions in asthma attacks, emergency room visits, and lost fewer days of work or school.

Chapter 5: The Proper Diet and Exercise for Asthma

It is important to maintain a healthy and balanced diet when you suffer from asthma. Although there is no certain diet that you should follow, it is important to stay healthy because those who suffer from obesity tend to have more severe cases of asthma. By exercising regularly and following a proper diet, you can boost your chances of feeling healthy, energetic, and full of easy breaths. This chapter will explain what kinds of foods are best to include your diet for treating asthma symptoms and it will also cover some great exercises that you can perform if you have asthma.

Coffee

People have used coffee as a natural way to treat asthma since the nineteenth century. You've probably heard how much coffee is bad for you in all other areas of health, but in this instance, coffee is on your side. Coffee is effective in treating asthma because the caffeine in it helps your airways stay open and can keep you from wheezing. Studies have shown that those who drink coffee have a third less chance of developing asthma symptoms. Many doctors recommend only drinking three cups to get the maximum benefits and you should never give coffee to children with asthma.

Onions

Onions are an excellent food to include in your diet because of their great anti-inflammatory properties. There are even studies that have shown that onions can help open up your airways during an asthma attack. To help reduce your chances of having an asthma attack, it is better to eat cooked onions instead of raw. Onions are easy to include in your diet and they're a healthy vegetable. You can add onions to salads, sandwiches, and soups.

Hot/Spicy Foods

Hot or spicy foods can be excellent for opening your airways. In particular, peppers stimulate special fluids to form in our mouths, lungs, and throats, which in turn loosens mucus and eases your breathing. Great examples of hot foods to eat for asthma are chilli peppers or anything with the spice Capsaicin. You can add peppers to your sandwiches and salads, or if you're feeling really brave, you can snack on them by themselves.

Foods with Vitamin C

People who suffer from asthma have low levels of vitamin C in their lungs. Vitamin C is an important antioxidant that lives in your bronchi and it can help reduce wheezing. To help control your asthma, you can incorporate plenty of

Vitamin C into your diet. You can give your body the right amount by drinking three glasses of orange juice per day or otherwise take 300mg of it in the form of a supplement. Some great examples of foods with Vitamin C are oranges, cantaloupe, red bell peppers, blueberries, broccoli, papaya, tomatoes, Brussels sprouts, and strawberries. Vitamin C is one of the easiest vitamins to add to your daily diet because it is abundant in many great foods and drinks.

Seafood/Fish

Fish are a great food to eat to help control your asthma because they contain omega-3 fatty acids. As you may recall from Chapter 3, omega-3 fatty acids help reduce reactions to asthma triggers. If you are able to eat seafood, try to eat plenty of salmon, tuna, sardines, and mackerel, all of which contain omega-3 fatty acids. Studies have shown that both kids and adults can cut their risk of having a severe asthma attack by eating these types of fish. Fish is great by itself with a healthy vegetable or on a sandwich.

Apples

By eating at least two to five apples per week, you can significantly reduce your chances of having an asthma attack. Researchers believe that flavnoids, which are compounds found in apples, can help keep your airways open. Apples make a great healthy snack and they're perfect if you're regularly on the move. You can cut them into slices or eat a whole one.

Carrots, Sweet Potatoes, Green Peppers

These vegetables can be helpful in reducing the occurrence of exercise-induced asthma. They contain an antioxidant that your body can convert into Vitamin A, which can help keep your airways open. These vegetables can serve as a great side dish, especially when paired with another asthma-healthy food such as fish. You can also add them to soups, salads, and sandwiches if you desire.

Garlic

Garlic is another food that contains an antioxidant called allicin, which works like a vitamin to decrease any free radicals in your body. Garlic is an anti-inflammatory food, too. Many people have regarded garlic as a top remedy for many ailments and illnesses for centuries. Garlic is a good spice to add to most of your food.

Milk

Since milk contains plenty of Vitamin D, which reduces free radicals in your body, it can be helpful in relieving asthma symptoms. Milk is a great breakfast drink and you can also add it to your coffee, cereal, or oatmeal. However, it is important to find out if you have a milk allergy before drinking it to ensure that you don't worsen your asthma symptoms with an allergic reaction. Milk allergies are one of the most common food allergies, as I will discuss in a few paragraphs.

Avocados

Avocados can be helpful in relieving asthma symptoms because they contain an antioxidant called glutathione, which also protects your body against free radicals. Avocados are easy to include in your diet because you can add them to salads, tacos, crackers, guacamole, and other delicious dishes. You can even cut one open and eat it right from around the core with a spoon.

Allergy Reminder

If you know that you are allergic to a certain food, take extra caution to avoid eating it directly or eating foods that contain it. If you have an allergic reaction from eating something, you could trigger an asthma attack on top of it. The most common types of food allergies that affect adults are milk, peanuts, shellfish, and eggs. If you are allergic to any of these food products, you should avoid foods that contain them at all costs. If you suffer from asthma but you are unaware of having any food allergies, it can be a good idea to see an allergy specialist to make sure that you don't have any. If you do have a food allergy, always make special requests when dining out and always read the labels on food products before buying them.

Exercising With Asthma
Exercise is important to your health and body because it helps you stay strong, fit, and active. Almost every part of your body is positively affected when you exercise—not only do your muscles, joints, and bones grow stronger, but your lungs grow stronger, too. If you suffer from asthma, one of your treatment goals should be to learn how to maintain a normal and healthy exercise regime. Often times, people with asthma won't exercise enough, out of fear that they will induce an asthma attack. However, exercising can actually help your asthma—as long as you know how to do it.

Low Exertion Activities

Sports and activities that do not require long periods of physical exertion, such as volleyball, softball, or baseball, are a good choice for those who have asthma, since they do not consistently put a demand on your lungs and body. With these sports, you're only moving for a short period of time before you can stop and catch your breath. High exertion activities, such as running, basketball, or field hockey are not good options because you are constantly working your heart and lungs. Cold weather sports such as hockey, skiing, or ice-skating should also be avoided because your airways can be sensitive to cold air.

Swimming

Swimming is a great way to exercise because indoor pools provide a warm, wet environment and warm air usually doesn't bother your airways as much as cold air. Swimming is a great endurance sport that is great for your cardiovascular health and can help make your lungs healthy and strong. It is also a fun sport and you can bring your friends along with you. There are many kinds of ways you can swim for exercise. If you're just looking to swim for fun while exercising at the same time, you can do the freestyle stroke, which is when you swim however you want. You can also practice the backstroke, the breaststroke, or the butterfly stroke.

Yoga

Yoga is a great and popular method of exercise among asthmatics. Practicing regular yoga can help ease your asthma symptoms and need for medication by 43%. Since yoga is a relaxation technique, it can help you learn how to control your breathing as well. There are many kinds of yoga poses but some are better than others when it comes to asthma.

Savasana pose: lay down and keep your arms to your sides. Make sure your palms are facing up and are open. Shut your eyes, relax your jaw, and begin focusing on your breaths. Take slow, deep, breaths as you try to relax the rest of your body. Remain in this pose for five to ten minutes while breathing slowly and evenly. Check out this YouTube video by Yoga Journal, Corpse Pose – Yoga Journal Poses, to see how to do this pose.

Sukasana pose: sit Indian-style, using a towel for support if you need it. Place your right hand on your heart and your left hand on your stomach. Close your eyes and lift up your chest. Breathe slowly and evenly for five minutes. Check out this YouTube video by Yoga With Adriene to see how to do this pose, Sukhasana (The Easy Pose) – Yoga With Adriene.

Forward Bend pose: Stand with your feet hip-width apart and fold your body like a jack-knife, slightly bending your knees if needed. Close your eyes, let your body hang forward, and take slow, deep breaths. This pose is good for opening your lungs and airways. Check out this YouTube video by Yoga with Adriene to see how to do this pose, Forward Fold Yoga Pose – Yoga With Adriene.

Butterfly Pose: Sit down, press the soles of your feet against each other, and let your knees extend to the sides like the wings of a butterfly. Pull your feet in toward your body and hold your ankles together. Take a deep inhale and then exhale while bringing your body forward. Take five deep breaths while you are in this pose. Check out this YouTube video, Butterfly pose, Yoga, by Ekhart Yoga to see how to do this pose.

Straddled Splits pose: Flex your heels and sit with your legs straddled apart. Tighten your thighs and inhale while stretching your arms toward the ceiling. Breath out and stretch your hands away from your body. Take five deep breaths while in this pose. Check out this YouTube video by Zao Yoga to see how to do this pose, Deep Hip Opening for Straddle Splits and Legs' Flexibility in Frog Pose.

Bridge pose: Lay on your back with your arms at the side of your body. Bring your feet back and lift your knees until your feet are below your knees. Lift your butt off the floor while pressing your back into the floor, expanding your chest in the process. Stay like this for 30 seconds to a minute and then breathe out, bringing your body back to the floor. Check out this YouTube video, Bridge Pose / Setu Bandha Sarvangasana, Yoga, by Ekhart Yoga to see how to do this pose.

Breathing Exercises

By learning how to practice special breathing exercises, you can help yourself control your asthma better. Many doctors believe that those who suffer from asthma tend to breathe quicker than normal and through their mouths, causing cool, dry air to reach your lungs. This type of air is more likely to trigger an asthma attack. Breathing exercises can help you regulate the way you breathe and can help reduce your chances of having an asthma attack.

The first type of breathing exercise that you can learn is called Diaphragmatic breathing. To do this, you can either sit or lie down. Focus on your breaths as you slowly inhale. Make sure that your abdomen extends out as your inhale, not your chest. As you exhale, your abdomen should go back in. When you exhale, it should take twice as long as it did to inhale. For a visual aid on how to breathe this way, check out this YouTube video by CioffrediPT, Learn the Diaphragmatic Breathing Technique.

The second breathing exercise you can learn is called Buteyko breathing. This type of breathing helps those with asthma lower the rate and volume of their breaths. To practice this breathing exercise, sit up in a chair and relax yourself. Look up to the ceiling or sky and close your eyes. With your mouth closed, slowly and shallowly breathe through your nose. Slowly exhale until there is no more breath to exhale. Hold your breath for three to five seconds and then breathe normally. This YouTube video by Christine Byrne, Buteyko Breathing Method, can help you understand this breathing method.

The third breathing exercise you can learn is called Pursed Lip breathing. This method of breathing is useful when you are experiencing an asthma attack because it helps you push more air out of your lungs. To do this, slowly inhale through your nose. Then, through pursed lips (as if you were going to whistle), exhale twice as slow as you inhaled. For the best results, combine Diaphragmatic breathing with Pursed Lip breathing. For a great visual aid on how to perform Pursed Lip breathing, see this YouTube video by COPDTV, COPDTV – Pursed Lip Breathing Technique.

Chapter 6: How To Pick The Right Asthma Doctor

Although asthma is controllable, it is still a condition that needs special attention. It is important to have a good relationship with your doctor if you suffer from asthma. You must be able to communicate everything about your condition to your doctor so that you can keep your asthma symptoms under control and prevent severe attacks from happening. It is a good idea to schedule regular check-ups so that your doctor can monitor your health and catch anything that may end up worsening your asthma.

If your asthma is mild, your general doctor can probably help monitor your progress. However, if you do not already have a general doctor, or if you have severe asthma and are considering finding a doctor that specializes in asthma and respiratory issues, it is important to understand how to pick the right one. Remember to remind yourself that your health is of utmost importance and you deserve the best care possible.

The first step in finding the best doctor is to know what kinds can help you. If you think that your allergies are affecting your asthma, you can look into seeing an allergist, which is a doctor that is an expert in identifying and treating allergies. You can also consider going to an immunologist, a doctor that is similar to an allergist but specializes in identifying factors that affect your immune system. A pulmonologist is a doctor that specializes in treating your airways and lungs and can usually help you control your asthma.

Once you decide what kind of specialist you want to see, you can do an internet search for your region, check your local yellow pages, or ask anyone else you know who has asthma. Usually, one of the best ways to find a great doctor is to find one via word of mouth. If somebody you know had a good experience, you can count on having a good experience yourself. You can also check to see if your insurance company has a list of specialists who are in their network.

When you go to your doctors appointment, have a list of questions and concerns ready. During a typical visit to a specialist, your doctor should properly examine you to determine the severity of your condition. He or she should also help you set attainable goals to help you manage your asthma. He or she can also help you create or review your asthma action plan, in case you ever have an attack. If your doctor doesn't explain something to you, don't be afraid to ask questions. If he or she gives you an inhaler or nebulizer, make sure that you are given clear instructions on how to use it. It is the job of your doctor to be thorough, patient, and to answer all your questions as best as possible.

Conclusion

I hope this book was able to help you to learn a little more about asthma and how to get it under control using several different methods and strategies.

The next step is to think about how asthma affects your life so that you can take the necessary action to life a more enjoyable, easy-breathing life. Evaluate your home for asthma triggers, rethink your diet, consider checking in with your doctor to get the best medical treatment, and make some room in your schedule to exercise. Anyone with asthma can live a great, satisfying life by following the steps and strategies in this book. Now it's time to take a deep breath and get ready to live like you've never lived before.

Finally, if you discovered at least one thing that has helped you or that you think would be beneficial to someone else, be sure to take a few seconds to easily post a quick positive review. As an author, your positive feedback is desperately needed. Your highly valuable five star reviews are like a river of golden joy flowing through a sunny forest of mighty trees and beautiful flowers! *To do your good deed in making the world a better place by helping others with your valuable insight, just leave a nice review.*

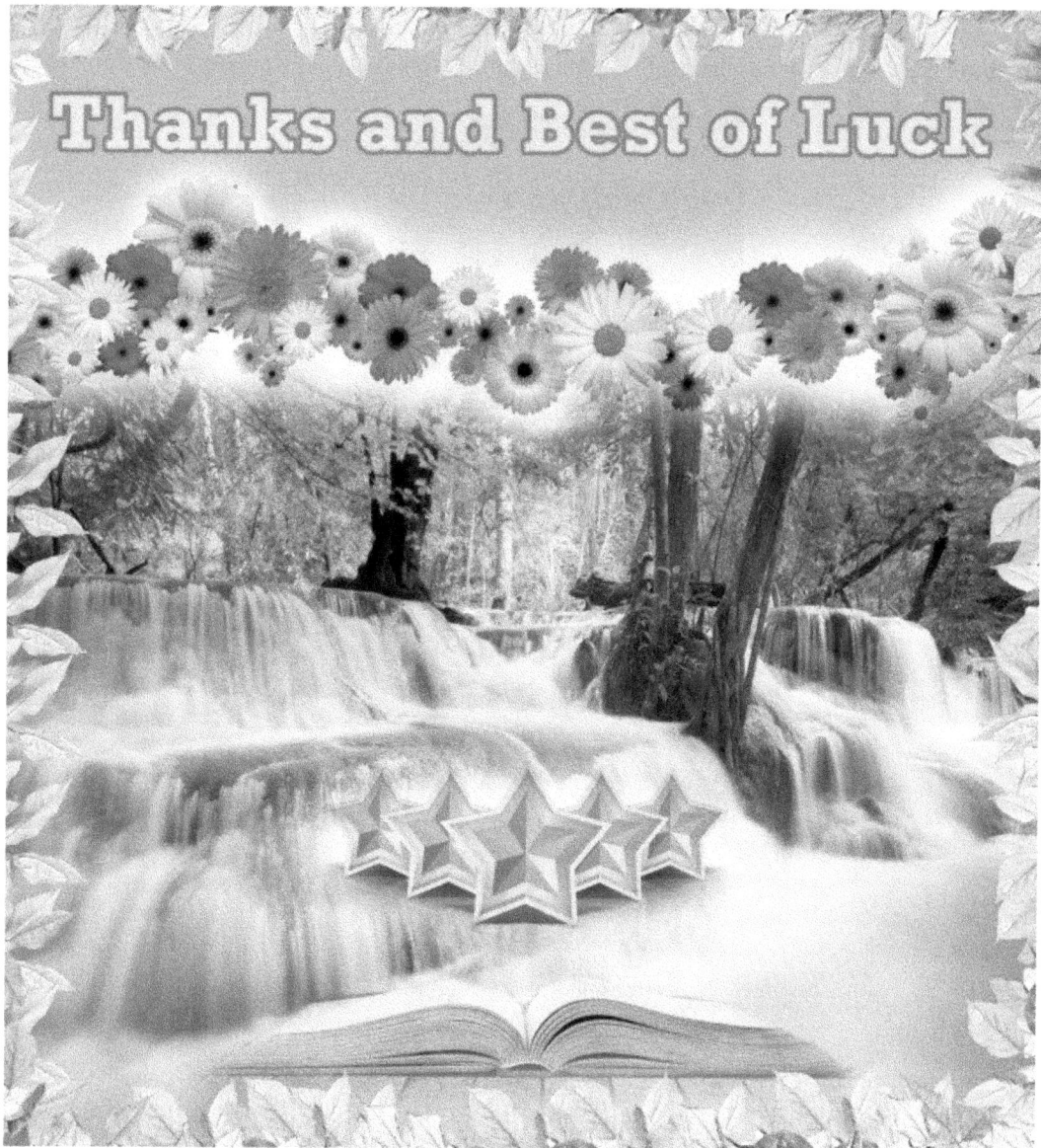
Thanks and Best of Luck

My Other Books and Audio Books
www.AcesEbooks.com

Health Books

ULTIMATE HEALTH SECRETS

HEALTH

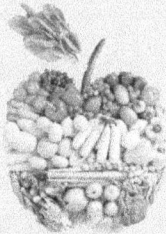

Strategies For Dieting, Eating Healthy, Exercising,
Losing Weight, The Mediterranean Diet,
Strength Training, And All About Vitamins,
Minerals, And Supplements

Ace McCloud

ENERGY
ULTIMATE ENERGY

Discover How To Increase
Your Energy Levels
Using The Best All Natural
Foods, Supplements
And Strategies For A Life
Full Of Abundant Energy

Ace McCloud

RECIPE BOOK

The Best Food Recipes
That Are Delicious, Healthy,
Great For Energy And Easy To Make

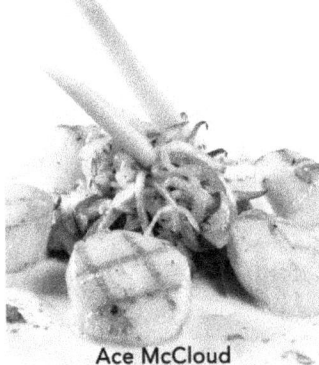

Ace McCloud

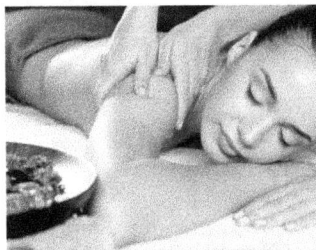

MASSAGE THERAPY

TRIGGER POINT THERAPY
ACUPRESSURE THERAPY
Learn The Best Techniques For
Optimum Pain Relief And Relaxation

Ace McCloud

LOSE WEIGHT

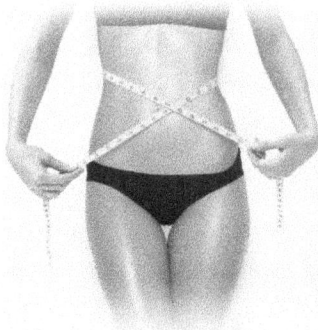

THE TOP 100 BEST WAYS
TO LOSE WEIGHT QUICKLY AND HEALTHILY

Ace McCloud

FATIGUE
OVERCOME CHRONIC FATIGUE

Discover How To Energize
Your Body & Mind So
That You Can Bring
The Energy & Passion
Back Into Your Life

Ace McCloud

Peak Performance Books

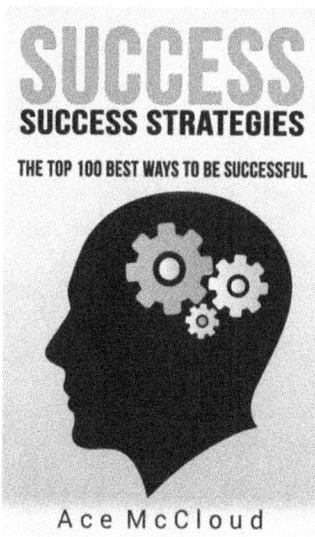

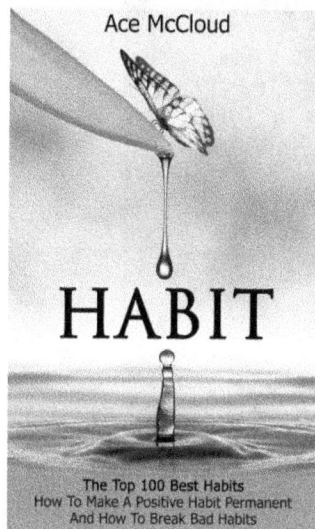

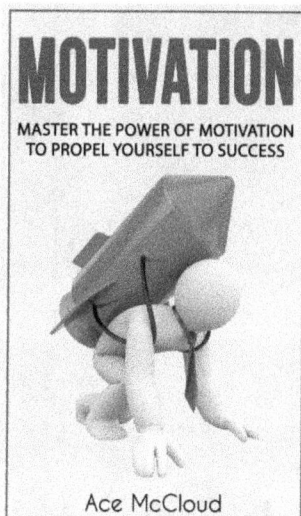

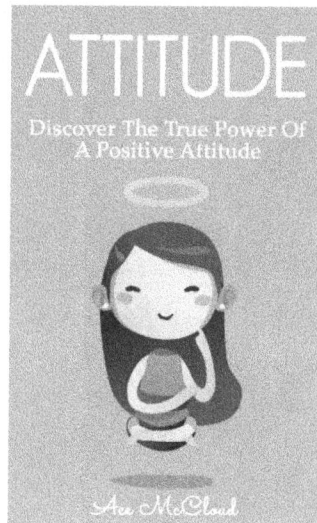

SUCCESS
SUCCESS STRATEGIES
THE TOP 100 BEST WAYS TO BE SUCCESSFUL

A c e   M c C l o u d

Ace McCloud

HABIT

The Top 100 Best Habits
How To Make A Positive Habit Permanent
And How To Break Bad Habits

MOTIVATION
MASTER THE POWER OF MOTIVATION
TO PROPEL YOURSELF TO SUCCESS

Ace McCloud

ATTITUDE
Discover The True Power Of
A Positive Attitude

Ace McCloud

SELF DISCIPLINE

Unleash The Power Of Self Discipline, Influence And Willpower In Your Life To Achieve Anything

Ace McCloud

Competitive Strategies

WINNING STRATEGIES

The Top 100 Best Strategies For Peak Performance During Competitions

Ace McCloud

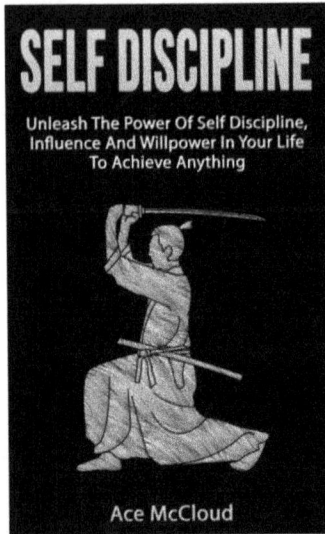

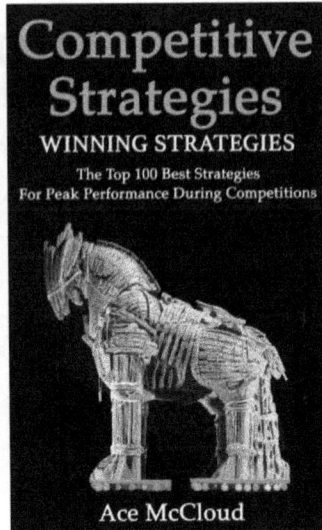

Be sure to check out my audio books as well!

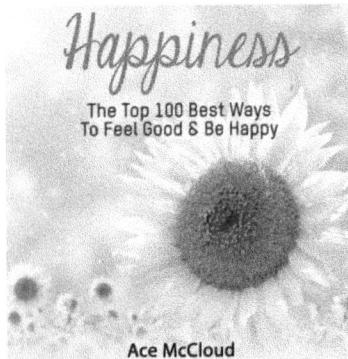

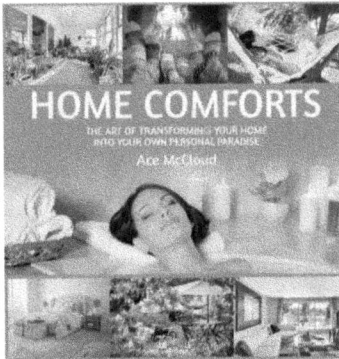

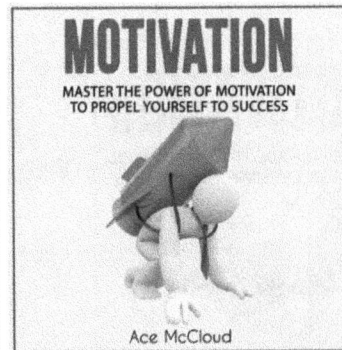

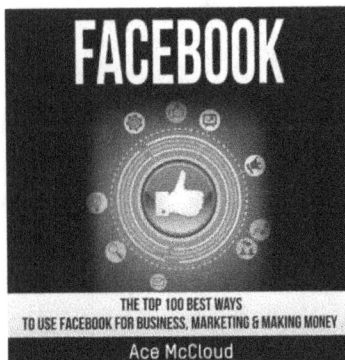

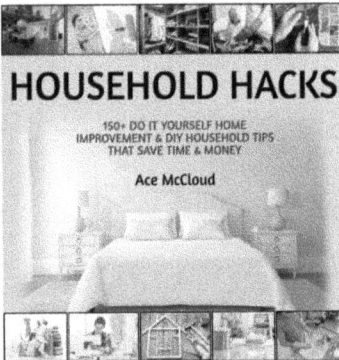

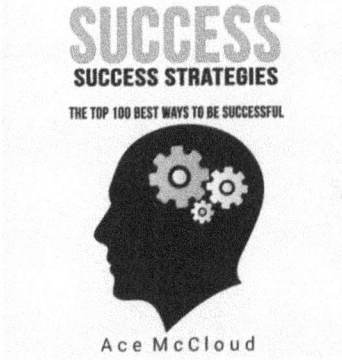

Happiness

The Top 100 Best Ways To Feel Good & Be Happy

Ace McCloud

HOME COMFORTS

THE ART OF TRANSFORMING YOUR HOME INTO YOUR OWN PERSONAL PARADISE

Ace McCloud

MOTIVATION

MASTER THE POWER OF MOTIVATION TO PROPEL YOURSELF TO SUCCESS

Ace McCloud

FACEBOOK

THE TOP 100 BEST WAYS TO USE FACEBOOK FOR BUSINESS, MARKETING & MAKING MONEY

Ace McCloud

HOUSEHOLD HACKS

150+ DO IT YOURSELF HOME IMPROVEMENT & DIY HOUSEHOLD TIPS THAT SAVE TIME & MONEY

Ace McCloud

SUCCESS

SUCCESS STRATEGIES

THE TOP 100 BEST WAYS TO BE SUCCESSFUL

Ace McCloud

Check out my website at: www.AcesEbooks.com for a complete list of all of my books and high quality audio books. I enjoy bringing you the best knowledge in the world and wish you the best in using this information to make your journey through life better and more enjoyable! **Best of luck to you!**

www.ingramcontent.com/pod-product-compliance
Lightning Source LLC
Chambersburg PA
CBHW080633030426
42336CB00018B/3181